Young, Dumb
&
Full of hmm...

By the Chapter

I. R. Wright

Young, Dumb & Full of hmm… is a work of nonfiction. Names and identifying details have been changed.

Copyright @ 2019 by TheraWrite, LLC

www.therawritellc.com

ISBN: 978-1-7336082-2-0 (ebook)

Author: I. R. Wright
Editor: Stella Samuel
Cover Design: x-potion designs

CONTENTS

C is for Chuck

—

Dating a much older man.

Reality Star Twin: Mark
Reality Show: *90 Day Fiancé*
Why him: Mark was dating a woman (Nikki) who was almost 40 years younger than him. During the show, he seemed more focused on protecting his finances than on bonding with his younger woman.
Similarities to him: The age difference between Chuck and I somehow made him want me to pay for everything. It was reverse sugar daddy-ism.

I was twenty-one when I met Chuck. He was thirty-three. I loved that a man so much older than me was interested in dating me. I believed it was proof of my maturity. Proof of my value as a significant other. I heard dating an older man was a gift. I understood they don't play games or waste time dating girls they aren't interested in. So, I believed dating an older man meant I might be graduating from dating and entering a realm of potential marriage.

I also believed older men were more financially stable. So, dating Chuck may have led to some very nice dates and dinners out. Mature experiences that would stretch my mind and help me see more than I would experience with a younger guy.

Teacher's Lounge

I met Chuck at a surprise birthday party for a former teacher turned mentor of mine, Stacy, in July 2005. Walking into the party I was nervous, worried I wouldn't have anyone to talk to. The only person I knew at the party was the birthday girl, and I assumed all her friends would ignore me since I was so young. It felt like walking into the teacher's lounge in elementary school. I knew I didn't belong in there and was afraid someone would kick me out. *"No kids allowed,"* they'd shout at me, even if they didn't kick me out.

Growing up, I was taught 'children don't speak when grown folks are speaking,' so I was also feeling that. Like, I wouldn't be able to talk to any of the party guests. Although, I had permission to be in the teacher's lounge this time, I planned to be seen but not heard.

My plan for the evening was to wait around until Stacy arrived, wish her a happy birthday and disappear while she worked the room greeting other guests. I loved her and wanted to show her some birthday love, but I had no interest in hanging out with her friends. I figured I could make it through the awkward times until she arrived. Since it was a surprise party, she arrived after everyone else. I was on my own until then and prayed she'd show up soon after my arrival.

The party was at a restaurant in Harlem. It was small and tucked in the ground floor of a residential building. Open, yet cozy and romantic, the dark room felt like a basement with a street view. Marc, Stacy's husband, reserved the restaurant for the night, closing it to the public. The only people in attendance were there for the party. Roughly forty people filled the small room. All eyes were on me when I walked in. It was exactly the kind of attention I was trying to avoid. They all looked for the birthday girl turning to face the door with excitement in their eyes until they realized I wasn't Stacy, then continued socializing with one another.

On the warm summer evening as the sun was setting covering Harlem's streets, cars and pedestrians with a soft orange glow, I walked into the restaurant past the bar to the right and mirrors to the left looking for a familiar face. I'd hoped to find another student, someone I knew wasn't older than me. Surveying the faces in a quick glance, I got stuck on one. His smile had me. I glanced past him then back to his smile again. That smile, that face was not a face I'd seen before. His face spoke to me. His mouth, soft and inviting, almost said, 'I don't bite.' I looked again, met his eyes, and was taken aback when he looked into mine. Without saying anything, his eyes said he was happy to see me. His cheeks raised in a wider smile as if to let me know he was hoping to spend some time with me, and his eyebrows arched inviting me over for just that very thing. For a second, peace washed over me. I belonged. Instead of getting caught in the teacher's lounge, I was in the school yard with a cute boy.

Chuck was a friend of my mentor's husband, Marc. We had immediate chemistry which created a magnetic force pulling us to one another through the crowd until we met face to face. I didn't notice Marc watching once Chuck and I were a few feet away from each other.

Forbidden Fruit

"Stay away from Chuck," Marc said in a serious yet playful tone. He didn't want to embarrass me, but I could tell he was serious. Marc was also a teacher and spoke to me as if we were in a classroom. He tried to lighten up and recognize we were in a lounge and not at school, but he was clear about this mandate. He looked at Chuck and back at me saying, "As a matter of a fact, you two stay away from each other." Marc watched us chatting and had to notice us flirting.

Looking at me he added, "Chuck is too old for you," before walking away to greet other guests. Marc's warning to stay away from Chuck because he was too old for me felt more like a challenge than a reason to walk away.

I knew I was mature enough to date an older guy, and my insides got a rise to prove it. Plus, Chuck was evidently interested in me. Well, I thought so anyway. Marc's warning gave me more confidence that Chuck was checking me out. Clearly, Marc saw something in his friend's disposition and behavior that affirmed Chuck's interest in me. I felt a sense of pride. This man, this handsome older man, was attracted to me. He was much older and likely accomplished, since he was friends with Marc – you know, birds of a feather. I knew Marc was very successful, hell he bought out a whole restaurant for his wife's birthday. So, this distinguished, much older man found me attractive. Challenge accepted.

What Had Happened Was

A friend of Chuck's walked over and interrupted our private conversation. I'd bet Marc sent that friend to interrupt our conversation and connection. I didn't want to look needy or be an awkward third wheel, so I backed up to let them talk. Instantly, I felt back in the teacher's lounge with no one to talk to.

Stacy still hadn't arrived, so I decided I would go to the bar and get a drink. If I was lucky, I might still get a chance to talk to Chuck once he wrapped up his other conversation, but I wouldn't push. I hoped he'd come find me.

A drink called *What Had Happened Was* intrigued me. It sounded delicious though it may have been an omen for what I would say later to explain the rest of the night with a drink of something tall, dark, and handsome. Of course, I ordered it.

The *What Had Happened Was* drink was a combined concoction of different dark and light liquors. Anyone who drinks knows combining dark and light liquors is a terrible idea. Some liquors were infused with flavors like coconut and pineapple. Others were straight liquor. After several pours of various liquors, the bartender added a combination of rum and vodka with just a touch of juice. Despite my better judgement, or to be sure I would loosen up and relax, I sipped for a few moments before walking back to the tables where everyone was standing. It wasn't long before Chuck was back in front of me.

"What did you order?" he asked me.

"The *What Had Happened Was*," I said.

"How is it?" he asked.

"Very good. I was feeling it with my first sip," I said giggling with a big smile. Between Chuck and my new drink, I was almost high. The high kind of high falling in love gives… Love, lust -- it all feels the same at first, right?

"Oh really? I need to order one. After I finish this one," he said holding up his drink.

We talked more and got to know each other a little better. He asked me, "How do you know Stacy and Marc?"

"Stacy was my teacher in high school," I explained. Our conversation was nothing of substance, just small talk. The drink was delicious. My shoulders relaxed. I stood a little taller with my head held high. Confidence found in a drink or the attention of a nice looking man radiated from me.

Stacy arrived a short time later, and everyone sat down to dinner. Although my initial plan was to leave upon her arrival, I had a new reason to stay. Plus, the place was so small, there was no way I could sneak out. I didn't want the trouble of explaining myself or why I needed to leave. Deciding to stay, I found an empty seat and sat down. I chose a wall seat at a four-person table. Two seats were on the wall and the other two were individual chairs on the opposite side of the table. I hoped Chuck would follow me, so I searched not just for an available seat, but an empty table. I preferred the cushion of the bench beneath me and coziness of the padded wall behind me. Plus, I was sure Chuck could identify me faster if I faced the crowd rather than with my back to the crowd. I was thrilled when Chuck followed me to the table and sat down across from me. *Jackpot!*

Two ladies sat down at the table with us. They both knew Chuck, but I did not know either of them. I finished my drink shortly after sitting. There was no way I would vie for Chuck's attention with two other women but I hoped he'd give it to me generously.

Being at the table would require more relaxation and confidence, so I waved to get the waiter's attention to order another drink. Despite having two other people at our small table, we continued to flirt with one another. We tried to use discretion as things between Chuck and I accelerated. *What Had Happened Was* may have been the culprit, but I didn't complain.

I ordered another drink for myself and one for Chuck. I hesitated because I would have preferred him buying me a drink instead. But I wanted to show him right away that although I was younger, I was able to hold my own and could easily afford to buy him a drink. It also put me in the driver's seat. *I might be young, but I'm not afraid*, was the message I was trying to send him. *I am bold. I am brave. I am mature. I can handle you.*

With each sip of our drinks we exchanged pieces of our inhibitions for courage. Within a few sips, any reserve still lingering from my pseudo-teacher's lounge sensation was gone. In fact, we had moved quickly from the lounge to the school's playground to my mom's house with no one home, figuratively.

Chuck and I touched under the table, holding hands and playing footsie, smiling at each other. We simultaneously managed to engage the two women at our table in conversation. We acted like a couple who arrived at the party, possibly together, to have our own date night. We did not act like two strangers who had only met moments before. Strangers who didn't know anything about one another. Well, anything other than our first names. Our physical energy grew with every sip of those drinks. Each sip brought us closer. The more we drank, the more we acted as if we had known each other for much longer than we had.

After that first sip together, we felt as if we'd known each other for a week. And after the second sip, we had known each other for a month. Half way through the drink we were acting like friends or maybe even lovers for years before we each walked into the bar that night. The level of comfort and connection was uncanny. I would love to believe I would have not been so open with him without the drinks, but the facts are the facts. Through all this we continued to engage in conversation with the other two diners at our table but still shared private interactions under the table. But when Chuck locked eyes with me I may as well have been the only lady in the room, much less at the table.

We ate and talked while touching in secret under the table all night until it was clear the party was over. Guests got up out of their seats and gathered their belongings to head home. I hated what was next. With the party over, I had to leave. I had to say goodbye to Chuck. It was all too soon. I couldn't imagine where the time had gone and wanted to be back at the beginning of the night with time to spend with Chuck all over again, but it was time. I needed to protect my image and didn't want to be the last to leave. Even if in truth I wanted to stay and have more time with Chuck.

After a bit of thought, there was no way for me to get around the facts. Everyone was up out of their seats mixing and mingling when I told Chuck I was about to leave.

"Okay, well, I definitely want to keep in touch with you," he said.

Whoooohooo! I'm sure my face said, and I couldn't have been happier. Marc's warning to stay away from each other held no weight until that point, and it would not stop us from moving forward and getting to know each other. Still, we wanted our connection to be our little secret.

Given the size of the place, everyone would have seen us writing on napkins or pulling out phones to exchange numbers. There was no way we could remember each other's phone numbers after so many drinks. We devised a brilliant plan to exchange numbers outside. The plan comprised of me walking outside first after saying goodbye to Stacy and Marc. Chuck would then follow behind. I liked the idea of having a few more private moments together before we parted. Any excuse leading to time together was perfect.

PDA

Once outside, I walked a few buildings away from the restaurant to wait for Chuck. When he arrived, he didn't ask for my number right away. Chuck offered to walk me to my car a few blocks away to be sure no one saw us exchanging numbers. *What a gentleman,* I thought. "I'd love that. Thank you," I said as I turned to start walking. It was nice having a gentleman walk me to my car late at night in the city. I smiled as we walked and thought, *He's smart. It makes sense. Let's be safe and get further away from the party before we exchange numbers.*

"Here's my car," I said. I didn't get a chance to unlock the door. Chuck pulled me close to him and kissed me with the same passion I'd seen earlier in the restaurant. Right there on the side walk, he leaned in wrapping his arms around my body. I was safe in his arms. Comfortable. And incredibly turned on. I don't know how it started, but we couldn't get our hands and lips off one another. I enjoyed the moment, the kiss, and his hard body against me before my conscience kicked in nagging me. It was terrible timing. Instead of yielding to and enjoying the moment, I worried about what we were doing on a busy Harlem street. Anyone could drive by and see us. Like, heaven forbid, my dad, or one of my dad's friends or someone from the after-school program. I closed my eyes and took a deep breath trying to calm down my inner good girl and get back in the moment thinking. *Just relax. No one can see my face since it's smashed into Chuck's.* After calming myself, I returned to the moment and enjoyed Chuck's lips again.

There I stood on a sidewalk in Harlem making out with a handsome guy. What luck I had. I didn't want to leave. I wanted to stay wrapped in his arms. *Yes! He really likes me. This is wonderful. He likes me as much as I like him. He likes me so much that he's willing to make out with me out here on this busy Harlem street.* Then I realized this incredibly deep public display of affection was occurring on a New York City street.

My conscience kicked in again. In the inner good girl versus inner bad girl fight, I wasn't sure which would win. I started thinking again, *What if someone recognizes my car. They'll know it's me for sure standing here…* before I got swept back up in the moment. My clear-headed, good girl side was no match for the enjoyment of making out with Chuck. We stayed in that spot making out for more than thirty minutes. Bad girl won.

My need to hide my bad girl ways returned again, aware of traffic driving by and wondering who might see me making out with this man, was ready to stop. Chuck pulled me back into the moment running his hands through my short afro. We didn't take a break or think to pause. All the tension built up between us at the restaurant, not to mention the added gasoline in the form of alcohol. *What Had Happened Was* indeed.

After a few hours of sensual tension, we unleashed and fueled our passion with another. Our heads moved to the left and then to the right as we hugged our bodies close. My conscience kicked back in, and I pulled my body away, but only just enough. I didn't want it to look like we were having sex. My face didn't move from his. My lips stayed connected to his as we kissed without pause. Chuck, having sufficiently released his tension from the party but still wanting more, placed his hands on my face and pulled me away from him. He looked into my eyes with sincerity.

The Invitation

"How do you feel about coming to hang out with me at my place?" he asked.

Breathing a happy sigh of relief, I said, "That sounds like fun." I did not want to leave him yet and was happy to receive the invitation.

"I'm going to go back inside to say goodbye to everyone," he said. "Stay here, and I'll drive around so you can follow me back."

"Okay," I said, finally making my way into my car.

"What's your phone number?" He remembered to ask before going back in. "Just in case I need to call you while we're driving," he said. I gave it to him, and he called me so I would have his.

Physically, Chuck was my type. He was tall, dark, and handsome. Warm, luscious chocolate skin tones like Djimon Hounsou's often made me lose my mind and good judgement. As in the case with Bobby, this instance with Chuck and with additional men I dated later.

Brown skin calls me like liquor calls alcoholics, and I get sucked into it. Confused by it. I get hypnotized looking at it. It might not necessarily be good for me, but it feels more than good at the moment. I have reflected on many relationships with dark-skinned men and realized they had me before they even tried. I am that weak to that complexion. I know it.

This delicious chocolate, I mean the taste of Idris Elba in all his beauty, that skin tone does something to me physically. It makes me happy. The way seeing someone smile causes you to smile. Or the way yawning is contagious.

Chuck had a broad muscular chest that reminded me of an ironing board in the best way. His arms begged 'hug me.' His presence made me feel safe. He had a head full of jet black curly hair which also covered his face through his beard and mustache. While I am more of a fan of low cut Caesars, he wore his cut well.

If I had taken a moment to think about Chuck's invitation to go to his house, I might have considered the likelihood of us having sex. I mostly focused on being with him. Otherwise, I wasn't thinking much at all. Caution completely thrown to the wind and flying high somewhere over Manhattan or maybe even in New Jersey by the time we decided to go home together, I didn't want our time to end.

Chasing the elation meant following him to his place. There was no concern about my safety. I knew people who knew him after all. I didn't worry about stopping myself from having sex with Chuck. I wasn't worried we had only met a few hours before. After waiting six weeks before having sex with Bobby, I understood waiting would not ensure a better outcome for any relationship.

As I waited in my car for Chuck to return, I looked at my phone to store his phone number and saw a bunch of text messages and missed calls reminding me I already had plans. Enzo, who I had been seeing before I met Chuck, and I had plans. I completely forgot. Remember, my evening started with the goal of leaving the party early, but *What Had Happened Was* happened, Chuck happened, and I wasn't about to let the night end.

I liked Enzo, but he didn't have the impact Chuck had over me. In that moment looking at my phone, I was far more intrigued by my possibilities with Chuck than what I knew Enzo could offer. Totally smitten with Chuck, I wanted to keep going with our fun conversation and physical exploration.

Right there waiting for a man I'd known for only a few hours and made out with for the past thirty minutes, I decided to cancel my plans with Enzo. As I thought about how to tell him my plans had changed, Chuck pulled up next to me. It was time to go. I would figure something out to tell Enzo, but another time. After confirming I was ready, Chuck pulled away from my car. If I wanted to spend the evening with him, I needed to follow. I gave my phone one more glance and drove away.

Within minutes of following Chuck, I lost him. I was convinced he went the wrong way up a one-way street to get on the bridge. I tried to call him in a panic, but I needed to drive. I wouldn't risk getting into a car accident, so I didn't follow him. I drove to my house. Once Chuck realized I wasn't behind him, he called me.

"Hey, why'd you stop following me?" he asked.

"Because I didn't want to die, and you drove up a one-way street the wrong way," I said.

"No, I didn't," he responded. "Anyway, do you still want to come over? I can come pick you up."

"Yes," I said and gave him my address.

Debauchery

I drove home and parked my car. Just then, I realized I had a major problem. Enzo. I had forgotten all about him and canceling our plans for the evening. Enzo lived close, and Chuck was headed my way. Enzo's building shared a driveway with my building. Chances were high Enzo would see Chuck and me. I was stuck, unsure what I should do.

Enzo's building and my building had entrances that faced each other. In between both buildings was a two-lane driveway, which led to the street. Sometimes people parked in the driveway for convenience if they were unloading groceries or running upstairs quickly. That would shut down one of the lanes and create a bit of traffic if cars were flowing in and out of the parking lots. There was a large parking lot for the tenants in Enzo's building just past our entrances on his side of the block and there was a smaller parking lot for the tenants of my building on my side.

Enzo and his friends would often hang out in their parking lot which had a clear view of the driveway, our parking lot and my entrance. Sometimes, they would hang out in the driveway. I didn't have a parking spot in our parking lot. so I always parked on the street. Once parked, I would need to walk through the driveway to get into my building likely running into Enzo and/or his friends.

My first thought was to avoid going into the driveway all together. I could park outside on the street and stay in my car and have Chuck pick me up there. But if Enzo came outside walked through the driveway and came to the street, he would still see me. My mind reeled... *What would I do if Enzo is at my car talking when Chuck pulled up? Maybe I should go inside.*

There was only one way for me to get inside, I would have to walk through our shared driveway. *But what if Enzo was outside in the driveway and I see him as I walk in? He would stop to talk. He'll question me about not returning his calls or texts. What would I say to him? I didn't get them. No. That's a lie. He would know I was lying. I didn't want to hurt him.* I needed to decide, and all my options were terrible.

Enzo was waiting to hear from me. Nothing I could say would justify seeing me with someone else. I wanted to go inside to freshen up before Chuck came, but I didn't know how far away he was or how much time I had before he arrived.

I called Chuck. "Where are you?"

"I'm still driving on the highway. I'll let you know when I'm outside," he said.

I needed his exact location but didn't want to appear desperate. "Okay," I said. Not helpful. Based on his highway location, I figured I had time, so I went inside. I wanted to freshen up, to have a look at myself. After the evening we'd had, I had to check my hair, my teeth, make sure I was still cute, and maybe even cuter if I had time, to be sure our night went well.

I still didn't know what to say if I saw Enzo. I didn't want to lie about canceling on him because I met another guy. I prayed quietly but aggressively to not see Enzo as I walked inside. *Please, God. Please, God. Please, God. Don't let me see this guy.* I didn't want Chuck to see us talking when he arrived, and I had nothing to say for myself. No excuse for ignoring him. No reason why we wouldn't be going out as planned. I walked faster and looked around hoping he wasn't outside. Praying hard not to see him and thinking about how I could quickly freshen up before Chuck arrived took all the mental energy I could muster. I couldn't think of anything to say to Enzo if I ran into him. My focus was on Chuck and looking my best for him.

Once I got in the building, I hurried. I walked fast while trying to look natural through the glass hallway leading to the driveway. I didn't want to run the whole way in case Enzo saw me. I wouldn't be able to make up an excuse for that. I had to look natural. So, I ran where there were walls and walked where he might see me through windows. My timeline was tight. I needed the transition to my apartment and back to Chuck's car to go smoothly.

I leaned my back against the door and sighed when I made it into my apartment. While leaning against the door, my cell phone rang. I froze then opened my bag, which had been resting on my arm, and fumbled through my things to find it.

It was Chuck. "I'm outside."

Dang, I thought. All that effort and he's here. I could still freshen up if I was quick. I didn't mind keeping him waiting, and he wouldn't mind a small wait, but I still worried about Enzo. He wasn't outside when I came in, so it was best to leave right away and not give him time to get outside.

"Where should I meet you?" Chuck asked.

I tried to think. "Umm… Come up the driveway," I said. *That was smart, right? The best option? In case Enzo was outside when I went back out. Right? Maybe not. Because if Enzo was outside, he might be standing next to the car. OMG. I don't know what to do. I need to get out fast. He wasn't out a moment ago when I came in so if I go out right now, he'll probably not be there.* The conversation I had in my head took longer than I had to give. I couldn't waste any more time.

I pulled my apartment door open and ran toward the stairs to make my way down the four flights. No time for elevators. I did the same fast walk past the glass windows in the hallway and made my way to Chuck's car relieved. *No sign of Enzo.* I didn't want Enzo to see me with Chuck, but I wanted to be with Chuck so bad risking it was worth it.

"Hey," Chuck said with a smile as I sat down in his car.

I smiled back. "Hey."

He put the car in gear and drove away. I was happy things had gone so smoothly and relaxed. But then, to my horror, I saw Enzo as Chuck drove out the driveway. Even worse, he saw me too. I didn't want to react and alert Chuck. Enzo looked at me with a smile as if I was about to stop the car and pick him up. Maybe he didn't notice there was a guy sitting next to me in the driver's seat. My eyes grew big as my mouth moved into a half smile. *Oops.* As we went past him, he mouthed a *whatthef-?* shrugging gesture. My eyes squinted into a weak apology as I waved back at him. We were off to Chuck's place.

I felt terrible. Disappointed in myself at a minimum. But also, because I knew I'd hurt him. I was 'Bobby-ing' this guy, and it didn't feel good. I took a deep breath and remembered who I was sitting next to. The guy I'd been trying to get closer to all night. With that sigh, I was over it and happy to see what the night had in store for me.

What Had Happened Was: In Progress

When we got to Chuck's, he was a total gentleman. He asked me to stay in the car then opened my door. Then, he opened all the other doors leading to his apartment for me to walk through. Once we were in his apartment, we had some casual conversation. I don't remember a single thing we talked about, but he was kind and polite. It didn't take long before we were back at it, like we had been on the street in Harlem. We were all about touching and kissing. Within a short time at his apartment, we made our way into his bedroom and on top of his bed.

Our passionate exchange continued, and Chuck climbed on top of me. He lifted my skirt but didn't take it off. As he moved my panties to the side, I thought about protection. *He wouldn't have sex with me without a condom,* I thought. I assumed he had put on a condom even though I didn't see him do it. *We were in his home. He probably had condoms all over the place and put it on discreetly when I wasn't looking.* My bad girl side wanted the passion and didn't want to ruin the moment, so I didn't investigate further. *Plus, even if he wasn't wearing one, he was safe, right?* He was Marc's friend, after all. That had to make him a cut above any average guy I might meet. I had so much respect for my mentor's husband, and I assumed his friends were respectable people as well. This guy was much older than me, so I also figured he was much more experienced with casual sexual interactions and would be certain to wear a condom. As I was thinking about whether he had wrapped it up and whether I should ask if he had, something unexpected happened.

My bottom jaw dropped in shock. In the darkness of the room, he couldn't have seen my face.

That was a good thing because I couldn't hide my surprise. His actions threw me for a loop taking me out of the passionate moment. *Yuck,* was all I could think. For no reason at all, he lifted my foot to his face and put my toes in his mouth. It gave me reason for pause to re-evaluate what I was doing there.

Wait a minute, I thought. *This guy puts toes in his mouth? This guy who I've been kissing almost nonstop for the past few hours. What?* To make matters even more yucky, it was summer, and I had been wearing sandals. I hadn't bathed or washed my feet since coming in from walking around in New York City. Gross. I mean, did Cinderella's prince suck her toes after he presented her with her glass slipper? I'm guessing *not.*

And worse, I saw for sure he didn't have a condom on. *Now, what?* I didn't feel comfortable asking him to put one on. He'd already entered me without one, so what's another stroke. *Right?* I'd heard if a man chooses to not wear a condom, it was a sign that he trusted his partner. He somehow found her special. She had the honored possibility of becoming his 'baby mama,' and he knew she was a cut above other women. As dumb as all that sounds, I did something dumber. I said nothing.

When we finished, we didn't speak about me going home. Despite some unexpected turns, I still enjoyed my time with Chuck, and he enjoyed his time with me as well. While still lying in his bed together, he wrapped his arms around me, and we fell asleep. I spent the night at Chuck's cuddling all night. I regretted my decision not to ask him to put a condom on. As much as I loved cuddling, I made every attempt to avoid kissing him remembering the toe-sucking display he'd performed not too long before. I felt special as we laid in bed together. With the attention and care he gave me all night, I enjoyed being with him despite fearing the consequences of what unprotected sex might mean.

Spilling the Beans

Chuck and I thought we'd used discretion sneaking out of Stacy's party. Our mistakes may have been drink related. The *What Had Happened Was* beverage death concoction may have been reason for our senseless thinking and behaviors.

"Hi, Miss Ivy," Stacy said after I answered my cell phone.

"Hola, Profesora. How are you today?" I asked.

"So, what happened between you and Chuck?"

Oh boy, I thought. *Just going to get straight to it, huh?* "Nothing," I said. "What would even make you ask that?"

"I know y'all thought you were being slick at my party, but you weren't. He made some stupid moves that caused me to pay attention to him, and I realized something was up."

"Huh?" I said trying to play dumb. I did not want to have this conversation. I tried to think of something to say to change the subject.

"What happened? You know I'm going to find out either way. Besides, if you're dating him, you need an older woman in your corner to protect you. Older men can be manipulative, and I don't want you to get hurt. So, tell me. What happened?"

I could not find a segue out of the conversation, and she kept pressing me until I spilled the details. Once Stacy knew about us, I felt the need to update Chuck. Marc and Stacy were his friends too after all, so I thought it fair to tell him what they knew about us. Since I was building a relationship with him, it was the right thing to do. I gave him an update after my talk with Stacy.

Chuck was not happy. His anger grew as he lectured me about why I shouldn't have told Stacy and how important his privacy is. We didn't talk for about a week after that call. He was upset with me, and I figured the relationship was over.

Despite Chuck's concerns and perspective, I had known my mentor for six years and had developed a bond of trust with her as well as a deep admiration for her. I loved spending time with her and looked forward to our phone calls and dinners together. She was a role model of what happiness was and she demonstrated a life I could aspire toward. I also knew she loved me as much as I loved her, and I valued her ability to care for me. So, while his reasoning made sense, it came down to her versus him. I had to choose which person I would be loyal to and have an allegiance with, and she and I had a proven history.

Stacy told me she felt responsible for protecting me. She didn't want me hurt in a relationship with someone so much older than myself, and she carried some personal liability because I'd met him through her. There was merit to that. She didn't want me to get played, or worse, get my heart broken. I didn't ask her why she thought he might break my heart, but maybe she knew about other relationships he'd been in. Her words echoed in my mind, 'Besides, if you're dating him, you need an older woman in your corner to protect you.'

The things she said made sense for the most part, so I decided I would keep her in the loop as I continued to date him. That didn't mean I would tell her everything, just what I thought I needed help with.

After my conversation with Chuck, I thought more about my conversation with Stacy. I reflected on the questions she'd asked and realized they didn't seem meant to help me. It was just information digging, like maybe she meant them for a third party. Possibly someone who had dated Chuck or was currently dating him. She asked questions she knew the answers to or could suggest answers for.

"Chuck's a very generous person, right?" She asked the question, but it was clear she knew the answer.

The questions she asked were too specific to his character. When I told her how sweet he had been opening doors for me, she said, "Oh, I'm surprised he was such a gentleman like that to you."

Eventually during our talk, I opened up to her. "I'm pretty sure he didn't wear a condom during sex."

"What?" she screamed. "He teaches sex education to help prevent HIV and AIDS, and he didn't wear a condom? What were you thinking? If he was someone else, we could be having a different conversation right now."

Overall, the conversation and the comments and back and forth didn't leave me with much confidence in the relationship I thought I was building with Chuck.

"You know he's not going to have a high level of respect for you since you had sex with him the first night you met him, right?" she asked.

Some comments she made were assumptions that didn't add up. For instance, she assumed he paid for the drinks we had at her party, but he didn't. I paid for them. That made me think maybe he wasn't that into me. If she assumed he'd paid for things, maybe it was because he did with girls he liked and he didn't like me much. Then, my thoughts switched to what Chuck said.

Maybe he was right. It might have been better to keep our relationship private. If I didn't tell her about our developing relationship, I wouldn't have to face judgement from Stacy or hear so much about what he usually does and doesn't do with girls. Those thoughts made me question our relationship as it stood.

The worst part of that conversation with Stacy when I reflected on it later was how I felt she was judging me more than helping me. Notwithstanding my actions of sleeping with a guy a few hours after meeting him, her comments cut deep.

I'd always thought she was someone I could confide in, judgement free, but after the conversation about me and Chuck, I felt different. It didn't destroy our relationship, but I was hurt. She'd always been someone I respected. Someone I felt achieved well. So, I considered what she said and had to toughen up to her criticism and take it with love knowing she was giving advice to help and not hurt me.

He Loves Me?

The foundation was shaky, but I liked Chuck. I liked who he was, what he represented, and the potential of us together. My birthday came and passed during our week of radio silence. He found out about it somehow and invited me over to his place to present me with gifts he bought me. There was a card, some bath stuff, and an erotica book. *An erotica book from a toe-sucker*, I knew it would be an interesting read. It was a pleasant surprise. Maybe he was into me? He was being generous as Stacy had suggested was typical of his behavior.

Chuck continued to make me feel special. He was sweet and thoughtful. One morning, after I spent the night at his house, I noticed the dress I planned to wear had a hole in it.

"Oh, no!" I said. I didn't have enough time to go home and get a new outfit without being late for work.

"What's the matter?" Chuck asked. I hadn't realized he'd heard me.

"There's a hole in my dress," I said trying to calm down. I tried to think of a way around the dilemma. *Did I have a sweater with me? Or at work?*

"Oh, don't worry I can fix that for you real quick," Chuck said. He pulled out a small travel sewing kit. "Keep getting ready, and I'll have this for you when you're done," he said with a smile. He wasn't concerned that he might be late for work. He stopped getting himself ready and focused on fixing my dress.

That small gesture showed he cared about me and demonstrated that by helping me. I also thought it was wonderful that he didn't shy away from sewing like it was only a girl thing. He did it without even thinking about it. He just didn't want me to worry.

Grinding

My preliminary focus when I met Chuck was my career. I knew I could have a great time hanging out with him or any other man, but I really wanted to get a full time job. I had been interning at *Essence* magazine when we started dating. Despite my love for spending time with Chuck, I was often more focused on my career. The idea of getting married kept moving further and further to the back of my head. The concept of what being in a relationship meant seemed even less important. I absolutely loved my time with Chuck, and that was enough for me. I didn't try to plan dates to hang out with him. We had spontaneous interactions. We would mostly get together when one of us realized we were in need of a hug or wanted some cuddling.

As a young intern committed to my profession, I tended to wake up to go to work at 5:00 a.m. and left the office around 10:00 p.m. So, sleepover dates were really the only kind we had. Sometimes I would get home early enough to have dinner with him, but that usually meant ordering take out and eating at his place. I was living with my dad during my time with Chuck. My dad never asked me where I was going or questioned what I was doing. I guess that's why I was able to live with him. He treated me like an adult, and I appreciated that. I needed that.

While Chuck seemed to love our sleepover dates, he hated my waking him up so early in the morning.

"What time do you need to be at work?" he asked me one morning when my alarm when off. It had woken him up.

"10:00 a.m." I responded.

"10:00 a.m.?" he said with pure annoyance.

"Yeah," I said confused at his reaction.

"So, why do you wake up so early? How do you commute in? Are you walking?" He asked half joking.

"Of course not," I said. "I go in early to get work done while it's quiet. I always have more work to do than time to do it in. So, going in early helps me get more done."

"It's really hard to get a good night's rest when you wake up this early," he complained to let me know I was disturbing his sleep.

To avoid the drama on the nights I slept over his house, I tried to wake up a little later so as not to disturb him. This annoyed me because I felt like he was taking me off of my grind. Asking me to go to work late meant I was going to be less productive in order to sleep or get more cuddle with him. At the time, it was more important to be at work. All things considered, I thought an hour was not too much of a compromise to have some romance in my life, but I stayed home when I wanted to wake up early.

In a gentlemanly fashion, Chuck always came out to meet me when I visited him at his apartment. He lived in a nice upper middle class safe neighborhood. I always felt comfortable around his place, so it wasn't necessary. However, I never resisted this seemingly sweet gesture. I would call him when I arrived, and he would come down stairs to let me in to his building and walk me upstairs to his second-floor apartment. I always thought this was one way he showed me that I was special to him. So special that he would leave his house to come and get me when he could more conveniently buzz me in. However, on more than one occasion, this proved to be a problem.

Fool Me Once

Everything was going great in our new relationship. Chuck and I never discussed our relationship status or exclusivity. We never had fights about needing to go out more or any major fights since the Stacy issue. We were both satisfied with what we were getting from each other. For me, hanging out with him was a refuge from my real life. Chuck offered a safe place for comfort and cuddles. That was it. There was no drama. Just happiness whenever we were together. It was perfect until one day in September 2005 about two months after we met.

That day, I had an unusual experience while attempting to enjoy a typical wonderful night with him. Before arriving at Chuck's house that evening, I called him to make plans to visit. As usual, he was happy to hear from me and welcomed my visit. When I arrived, I called him, as usual, so he could come downstairs to get me and walk me inside. This was his way of being a gentleman in a much welcome fashion. However, this time when the phone rang, I waited for him to pick up, but he didn't. It rang and rang until his voice mail picked up. *That's unusual,* I thought. No big deal at first. I waited with the phone in my hand certain he'd call me back right away. I had spoken to him moments before I left my place. My building was less than fifteen minutes from his, so I knew he was waiting for me, expecting my call. With confidence, I waited for him to see my missed call and call me back. At any moment.

In the meantime, I walked myself over to his building's front door. I didn't have to wait for him to come all the way out to get me. Even though he always did, I didn't need him to do it, especially if he wasn't ready yet. I made my way past the first glass door which was unlocked and was in the waiting area with several doorbells for each apartment. That's when it hit me. I didn't know his apartment number. I looked down at my phone and called him again. *Maybe he didn't hear the first one? Or was in the bathroom?* I tried not to justify being ignored, but I also didn't want to focus on the major detail of not knowing his apartment. I'd been inside. I must not have paid much attention. *So, this second call would let him know*

I am here because he totally missed the first one, I thought as his phone rang in my ear.

With each ring, my frustration grew. *How am I here, standing in lobby of his building and unable to get in, unable to press his buzzer because I don't know his apartment number?* It was crazy. His voicemail answered again, and anger washed over me. I knew he had a house phone, but I didn't know that number either. There I was outside calling Chuck again, unable to get inside.

I took a deep breath to calm down. I knew he would call me any minute, but somehow, the deep breath meant to calm me returned with rage from the possibilities. *Why wasn't he answering?* I was furious. *Is he in his apartment with another woman?* We were not an exclusive couple, so it wouldn't be terrible if he was seeing someone else. *But why invite me over if he had other plans?*

My mind ran laps trying to figure out what was happening. *Why wasn't he answering his phone? Why waste my time driving over here?* Beyond the drive, I'd also built up excitement over seeing him. The letdown was harsh. It was a long way down from the elation I'd had leaving my apartment to get to his. Worst of all was the idea someone else had taken my spot. Another woman might have been placed at a higher significance in his life than me. The inkling he would choose her over me, even though we had plans, was a gut check. A visit from this mystery woman wasn't planned, so the potential of him letting her into my spot hurt. I hated losing him to her and hated the feeling of embarrassment after showing up for someone who didn't show up for me, especially when I wasn't asking much of him to start.

Overnight dates were all we had. I had given him a lot of credit. He was sweet to come get me for our dates, but I didn't know exactly where he lived. I felt played in a game I didn't sign up to play. Certain he'd devised a way to stop me from interrupting a surprise visit from another woman by making sure I didn't know his buzzer number or house phone number, I was hurt and frustrated. Defeated and disappointed, I returned to my car and drove home. My safe place had been compromised.

Chuck did call me after I'd made it back home, had taken a shower, and was in bed. My phone rang, and when I looked at it, I was both angry and relieved to see his name. "I am so sorry," was the first thing out of his mouth. "Where are you?" he asked next.

I wrinkled my face in disbelief. He has some nerve asking where I was. "I'm home." It took everything in me to stop myself from ending that line with "Stupid." He knew I wasn't still at his apartment waiting to get in. "My phone was charging when you came over, and I didn't hear it ring. Can you come back?"

"Hell no!" I was pissed. But hearing his excuse, I believed it was a mistake. His tone felt genuine. I played tough, but I was happy he'd called. As angry and hurt as I had been before, I got over it once he apologized. I promised myself I'd get and remember his apartment number so I would never go through that again.

He Loves Me, Not?

Whenever I went to Chuck's place for our takeout dinner dates, he always asked me to pick up the dinner on my way in. That meant I was paying for it. He never offered to order food so it would be at his place when I got there nor offered to give me money once I arrived with the food. He always wanted the most expensive thing on the menu for our dinner dates often asking me to order things I'd never heard of before. When I did, the restaurants warned me they only make large servings, because of the unique order. I could afford to pay for the food, so I didn't mind too much, but I often made a mental note of it.

As time passed and Chuck continued this practice, I remembered what Stacy had told me about him before. He was a very generous person. It didn't feel very generous of him when I paid for all our dinners.

Maybe our relationship caused him to act out of character? If this guy is usually generous, why is he attempting to get me to pay for everything? Maybe he thought I was only with him for his money. From the very first night we met, I paid for things. So, that couldn't be it. Right? I didn't know how to explain his behavior. We went out as a couple one night to dinner and his behavior further demonstrated his financial concerns in our relationship. At a family chain restaurant, which I considered right up there with a drive thru, Chuck showed me once and for all how big a factor money was in our relationship.

I assumed Chuck would pay for the dinner when we sat down to eat. Given my own financial issues, I was happy to be out at a restaurant with him having dinner, but I was mindful of what I ordered. I didn't want to order anything too expensive because I hated the label gold digger. After we finished eating, the waiter brought the bill to Chuck and left the table.

"Why would he leave the check in front of me?" Chuck said offended. It left me dumbfounded. Not only did he have an issue with it, but he was so bothered by it he said something out loud. *Don't you have a job? He figured you wanted to be a gentleman and pay.* But I said none of that. He ranted on about why the waiter assumed he would pay. I couldn't believe how much fuss he made, but I let him vent.

His behavior that night made something I had been trying to ignore clear. I was the dominant financier of our dates. I don't know what bothered him so much about paying for meals. Financially, he seemed to be doing well enough. He owned two apartments and two cars. He was employed full time. No children, so no child support. No ex-wives, so no alimony.

The only rationale I could come up with for his behavior was maybe he had a sugar daddy complex. He knew how much older he was than me, and maybe it bothered him. Maybe he thought people around us figured I would only be with a guy as old as he was as long as he paid for everything.

Fool Me Twice

In February 2006, five months after the bad experience of not knowing which apartment belonged to Chuck while waiting for him to answer my call, seven months since we first started dating, history repeated. For a second time, after making plans to visit him, I showed up at his house, and he didn't answer the door to let me in. In an instant, my mind traveled back to the first time. A compounded anger built because I'd allowed myself to be in the same position yet again. It was infuriating.

I stood outside his apartment in disbelief. He didn't answer his cell phone. I called him several times back to back, nonstop until it hit me. He had no plan to answer. I left fuming. Beyond pissed. Not only had he done this to me, it was the second time it'd happened. Because I allowed it to happen again, I needed to take responsibility for this experience and realize I did it to myself.

And just like the time before, I was back home before he called me. I had no interest in answering his call. He called several times. Every time it rang, I hit the decline button and swore to never speak to him again.

A few days before this infraction was Valentine's day. I'd called Chuck on Valentine's Day expecting to spend time with him. He didn't answer and didn't bother to call me back until that day when we made plans to hang out. After blowing me off on Valentine's Day, I didn't expect he'd do it again. I was done. Chuck knew it too.

To rectify the situation, he left a voice message on my phone giving me his home phone number asking me to call him back. He said his phone was charging again and didn't want to miss my call. He almost got me. Men always give a little more when they know it's over. They know it and don't want their woman to leave. I was moved by the gesture, but I wouldn't give in this time. *Nice try*, I thought. *But, I'm done.*

I wanted nothing else to do with him. Over time and with all I had experienced in the non-relationship, I no longer had those good feelings I felt when I started dating Chuck. What I thought about instead were all the times I gave him credit for being a gentleman and coming down from his apartment to walk me in every time I visited. Each time, I'd decided was his manipulative way to keep me at a distance.

I didn't want to sleepover date him anymore. I didn't want to pay for our dinner dates anymore. Good riddance. Enough was enough. I said goodbye to what never was. Well… until life happened. I would desire his comfort again in no time.

Partyz 'n the Hood

The following night, Saturday, I had plans with a few of my girlfriends to go to a party in my neighborhood. The girls lovingly referred to it as a 'hood party. They explained that the party was usually a gathering for the people from the roughest parts of our neighborhood. I had never been to one of those parties and didn't know what to expect when I arrived.

Instead of being at a restaurant or a bar, this party was at a hall. The kind retirees rent out for dinners. There was no security when we walked in, just lots of people. Since it was a 'hood party, I wanted lots of security, police even. With metal detectors and guns. But I had no such luck. Instead, the entrance of the hall remained brightly lit which was weird for an adult party. But even stranger were all the people congregated in the entrance. There was plenty of room to move inside the actual hall, but many preferred to hang out near the door.

I find crowds nerve wracking. Walking through crowds is even more terrifying, so I was off to a horrible start. As I walked in alone through all the people, I scanned everyone around me for a familiar face. What I saw was beauty. All the guys and girls alike.

There were faces I recognized but couldn't place how I knew them. I wasn't sure if I should wave at them or not because I didn't know if I actually knew them from my past, like elementary school or if I'd just seen them in passing in high school. It would have been easy enough just to say hello regardless, but I thought, *What if they don't know who I am? I'd look weird waving at people who don't wave back.* Trying not to stare or appear lost, I checked out my surroundings and devised a plan. With bathrooms on the right and a dimly lit room towards the left, I headed into the dimly lit room. I assumed the party would be in there and I would find my friends. Fortunately for me, I saw them as soon as I walked in, posted up on the opposite side of the room at a table.

As if my, *do I know you or do you know me* dilemma and fear of crowds weren't enough, my discomfort raised when I saw both Bobby and Enzo in attendance. Bobby and I were long over at this point, but he still got a rise out of me. I cared about him, and I was devastated he was there because he acted like a different person than I knew him to be. He knew every pretty woman in the spot and was walking up and greeting them all, making them laugh like they were good friends. That was yet another eye-opening moment because I didn't know he had all these close female friends. He'd never introduced them to me while we were dating, and I hadn't seen them when we went out. To make matters worse, after looking me right in my eyes he acted like he didn't even see me. Like I didn't exist. That hurt.

Despite all the pain, embarrassment, and otherwise ridiculousness he put me through, I wanted him to acknowledge me in a loving way. I wanted to believe we were friends even though he did horrible things to me. The way he treated me felt like I meant nothing to him. It was all a game. And somehow, seeing him hurt me more than any of the bad situations I had been in with him prior. I put up a front for a while so my friends wouldn't know something was wrong, but inside, I screamed and cried. I expected him to give me a big hug. I thought he would finally admit I was the best thing he'd lost. But that was not the case, and I was a mess.

I was only at the party for an hour before I was ready to go. I'd gotten to the party at 1:00 a.m. and by 2:00 a.m., I'd had enough. I said my goodbyes and was gone. In desperate need of some repair from the distress, pain, and hurt I felt from my interaction or lack thereof with Bobby and wanting rid myself of those emotions, I called a friend while walking to my car. I told him I needed to talk because I was sad. He cheered me up. We talked while I walked to my car, the drive home, and as I walked into my building. I thanked him for being there and tried to settle in, but the pain worsened. I needed to feel better fast and with more impact than a simple phone call from a friend would bring. I wondered who to turn to. In the middle of the night, when I was feeling down, I knew who would be there in the ways I needed. The stress of the party led me right to Chuck.

After ignoring his calls and apologies for missing my calls when I showed up at his place the night before, I wanted to be with him. Then I stopped myself. I remembered I was done with him. But… I started making excuses again. *He did make sure to leave his house phone number this time… He was really sorry this time, and he tried to fix it.*

All things considered, I knew he could make me feel better. So, at 2:25 a.m. I made the call. "Hey Chuck."

"Hey, Ivy."

"Can I sleep with you?"

He didn't finish his short reply, "Of course," before I was off and running to the car. I didn't make it to Chuck's house with dry eyes. I cried hysterically the entire ride over. Bobby was horrible. Tears ran down my cheeks the whole way to Chuck's. Just ugly crying.

As I pulled up to Chuck's house, I hoped he would answer his phone. Still crying to myself while I parked, I called him to ask him to buzz me in.

"Dial 227," he said. And just like that, I had the house phone number and the buzzer. I wiped tears as I walked in. I ran up the stairs and rang his bell. My mood improved as soon as I saw him.

We sat down in the living room, and Chuck presented me with Valentine's Day gifts. A bottle of plum wine, a heart-shaped box of chocolates, a Valentine's Day candle, and a card.

Failure to Launch

Despite his sugar daddy complex and our lack of truly dating, I liked Chuck a lot. Our relationship was special. I compartmentalized it into a haven when I needed a break from life. We continued to date on and off for about two years, but I think the initial breach of trust with Stacy stopped us from ever really growing the relationship.

We spent night time dates using each other for cuddles and sex. We were both okay with it. The fact that I liked Chuck made the comfort of his presence effective. If I didn't like him, being with him would not make me feel better at all. His presence was calming.

Notwithstanding the intensity of our first sexual experience, our sexual tension didn't last. So much so, we phased it out of our relationship altogether. As time passed, we spent the nights together just cuddling.

Besides supporting my bad days with hugs in the bedroom, Chuck was someone I enjoyed calling on rough days at work. He would give me ideas on how to handle my office politics. I didn't listen to what he was talking about but talking to him soothed me. It was nice to vent about whatever bothered me. I often combined my venting with flirting, which helped shift my mood and attention. It was a win/win. Our conversations helped get my mind right and get back to work.

The Silver Lining

I don't remember how this relationship ended. With time, I found other ways to cope with my pain and the joy I felt instead of running to Chuck. I am thankful for my time with Chuck. He taught me that dating an older man would not make dating any easier or better. Thanks to this relationship, I do not use age as a pre-qualifier for any man I date or to determine if he will be the best guy for me. After Chuck, I dated guys I liked without a preference to older men. The last man I dated was six years younger than me, and I married him.

OKAY SO, HOW WAS IT? READY FOR MORE?

GET THE FULL BOOK SEARCH FOR:
YOUNG, DUMB & FULL OF HMM….

OR JUST THE NEXT CHAPTER:
- Dating a Police Officer
- Dating a Nerdy Nudist
- Dating a F- Boy
- Dating a Cute Thug
- First Teenage Love Affair
- Daddy's Love Lessons

Thank you for taking the time to read this Chapter! Was it what you expected? Something you think other people would enjoy?

I humbly and kindly ask that you please provide a review of this book. Share your thoughts to help others know what you experienced while reading this.

I am also looking forward to reading your thoughts.

PLEASE REVIEW THIS BOOK

ABOUT THE AUTHOR

I. R. Wright was married in 2017. She has one child and lives in a small town outside of New York City where she was also born and raised. This is her first book.

Join the Mailing List:

Irwright.com

Facebook.com/YoungDumbDating

Instagram: @YoungDumbDating

Amazon Author Page

Email: ivy@irwright.com